Yoga for E

Increase Your Flexibility and Fitness Level with Yoga

Nicole Harrington

Γ

Gamma Mouse

www.gammamouse.com

YOGA FOR BEGINNERS
Copyright © 2015 by Nicole Harrington.
All rights reserved.

First Edition: April 2015
1234567890
A Gamma Mouse eBook
Published by Gamma Mouse, a dba of Xilytics, LLC.
www.gammamouse.com

Introduction

Yoga came into my life at a point where I was getting increasingly frustrated with my decreasing flexibility. Things that I used to be able to accomplish suddenly became much harder, often leading to unwanted muscle aches and strain. The worst part was that my decreasing flexibility was starting to hinder the active life that I wanted to lead.

I tried various suggestions from friends, most of which revolved around a more active stretching program. The results were uninspiring to say the least. Then a close friend suggested I try yoga, that it not only helped them with their flexibility, but it also gave them an additional mental boost. Now many years later, I can say that the physical and mental benefits of yoga cannot be understated; it is truly one of the most incredible physical activities that we can do. Not only has it restored my flexibility, it has improved it, making me stronger, and less prone to strains and aches. I can't imagine living my life without it.

I am extremely happy that you have decided to learn about yoga, and the benefits it can provide for you. It is my goal to give you the general information and knowledge you will need to get started and to ultimately succeed.

So let's get started!

Limited Time Free Offer

Download the #1 Bestseller from Gamma Mouse Media for FREE! Hurry this offer won't last as it is for a limited time only. Reserve your free copy today at http://gammamouse.com.

Understanding Yoga

Yoga has long been known as one of the best ways to improve your well-being and overall way of life. There is a long list of benefits associated with yoga, but there are still so many people who are unsure about how they can get started.

Throughout this article we're going to give you an introduction to yoga; we'll explain the benefits, different yoga practices, and also let you know exactly how you can get started practicing yoga.

Benefits of Yoga

We're going to start by discussing some of the benefits of yoga—after all, chances are that you want to start practicing yoga because you want a healthier and happier life.

There are so many benefits of yoga and it really can be overwhelming for people who are just getting started. One of the most sought-after benefits of yoga is the fact that it can improve your overall health and wellness.

A wide range of yoga practices are available for you to take advantage of, with each one providing you with different benefits. The most basic practices can be used for meditation, whilst more advanced practices can provide you with more health benefits.

Different Yoga Practices

Many people who are unfamiliar with yoga think that there is only one style—there isn't. There are many different styles of yoga and these are commonly referred to as "practices". There are practices aimed at beginners and others aimed at people who are more advanced, so it is quite important for you to have an understanding of the different practices out there.

We won't go into too much detail on the different practices, but here is a short list of some of the most common ones you'll find:

Hatha

Kundalini

Ashtanga (sometimes referred to as "Power Yoga")

Vinyasa

Bikram (sometimes referred to as "Hot Yoga")

If you're a beginner, Hatha is generally the best practice to start with. It's a slow and gentle form of yoga that provides beginners with a solid foundation.

How to Get Started

One of the best things about yoga is that there are many ways to practice, you can take advantage of online learning courses, videos, DVDs, or even visit a yoga center if you want the best experience.

Firstly, think about which yoga practice you'd like to do—as mentioned above, we recommend Hatha. Then, think about how you would like to do this (i.e. videos, online learning course, yoga center).

A yoga center will generally provide you with the best experience and learning situation, but it also means that you have to commute to and from the center, and it can also be more expensive. You should weigh up the pros and cons of each method.

A lot of people think that yoga is all about practicing poses and stretches, but it's actually much more than this. As you can see, there are a lot of different yoga practices, some for beginners and others for those who are more advanced.

Hopefully you now have a good introduction to yoga and understand why it's so beneficial. Make sure to pay special attention to the "How to Get Started" section to find out how you can get started with yoga and progress onto the more advanced yoga practices.

How Yoga Can Help Your Health

To define Yoga in its original ancient Indian context can be quite complex since it is viewed as a science. This perception makes Yoga a way of life. However, in the modern world the basic understanding of Yoga is physical exercise that involves different body postures, breath control and meditation that helps in relaxation and body health. But how does Yoga help in general body health? I know that is a question that needs answers especially to newbies since yoga is mostly associated with meditation which has almost nil connection to body health. Don't worry. By the end of this article the "how yoga helps your health" concept will be demystified.

Yoga helps your health in the following ways:

Removal of toxins from the body. This is achieved through sweating.

Flexibility and strength training that aims at improving the inside body as well as the outside body.

Improvement of posture that results to alleviation of pain associated with the back, neck and shoulders.

Due to the stretching involved in Yoga digestion is put on track. This relieves acid reflux, constipation and irritable bowel syndrome.

Physical stamina is improved by holding postures in order to extend breaths.

The body gets a leaner and longer look resulting from the lengthening of muscles due to holding of postures and stretching.

Prevention of arthritis and disability mitigation. This is because you take your joints through a full range of motion when practicing Yoga. The full range joint movement prevents cartilage and joint breakdown,

Protects the spine. A balanced Yoga asana practice helps to keep the spinal disks supple. These disks are responsible for protecting the spine.

It betters your bone health. This is achieved through weight-bearing exercises practiced in Yoga and also through lowering of the stress hormone called cortisol that affects calcium in bones.

Helps in blood circulation by increasing blood flow and getting oxygen to your cells.

Decreases dangers of getting a heart attack or stroke by increasing your heart rate. Yoga achieves this by boosting levels of hemoglobin and red blood cells that carry oxygen to tissues.

Yoga helps to reduce blood pressure.

It reduces blood sugar by lowering adrenaline and cortisol. Helps in weight loss. All these in the long run significantly reduces the chances of complications like blindness and kidney failure.

It lowers stress level and improves depression by reducing cortisol levels.

Yoga maintains your nervous system. Yogis can easily induce heart rhythms, raise their hands' temperature as well as generate particular brain-wave pattern.

Yoga aides in getting good deep sleep due to relaxation mode the body switches to after engaging in Yoga practices. We all know that a person who slept well wakes up healthy, rejuvenated and ready to handle any task ahead of them.

It boosts body immunity. Some of the practices, for instance asana, meditation and pranayana improves immunity by boosting antibody levels when needed and reducing the antibody whenever necessary.

The lungs get enough room to breathe through Yoga.

There you have it! I have outlined how Yoga helps your health. It is now clear that you can keep away diseases and keep healthy through yoga practices.

Yoga as a Stress Reliever

Modern science has become more than instrumental in explaining how our bodies work. This has become one of the most beneficial ways of explaining how the holy practice of yoga is a crucial form of exercise that can be used to relieve stress; thus bringing or rather elevating that inner peace within our bodies. Yoga is rightly considered as a complementary physical exercise and mental discipline, which helps in achieving peacefulness of the mind, body and relaxation, thereby helping in managing stress and anxiety. With different types of yoga currently available, it becomes a personal preference in choosing the type of yoga that you feel works best for you in managing stress and anxiety levels. For instance, I personally prefer a type of yoga known as Hatha yoga, which has become vital in helping me manage stress and anxiety. On this note, here is how yoga can relieve stress in a holistic and scientific way.

How Our Bodies react when we are stressed

When bringing stress into context in a scientific way, it mostly revolves around the excess release of hormone cortisol into our bodies, thereby making the brain to work under pressure. This may be as a result of strict deadlines, lack of job, economic difficulties or any other thing that may lead the body to undue pressure. Knowing very well that high levels of stress can be so adverse to an extent of causing ulcers, weight loss, whacking out your immune system, or leading to high blood pressure, it is always advisable to incorporate yoga into your life. It is a simple and proven way of managing and relieving stress through following very simple body movements.

Using yoga as a way of relieving stress is based on harnessing our breathing patterns while slipping our bodies into a state of rest and digest. This will not only help our bodies in getting some relief, but also in returning our bodies into the normal state. This is done by lying down either on the floor or on the bed, while peacefully closing your eyes. This is followed by peaceful inhalation, which will enable the breath to expand the lower part of the belly then into the ribs and chest. The process of exhalation calls for the need of letting all the breath come out as it wants without any control, but just naturally. This pattern can be repeated in intervals of five minutes and will obviously work magic in relieving stress.

As noted above, incorporating the Hatha type of yoga in your daily routine is probably the best way of managing stress in your daily life. Its slower pace and easy body movements become even more advantageous to yoga beginners. Some of the benefits of incorporating such type of yoga in your daily life revolve around decreasing tension and stress, increasing flexibility, improving strength and balance, lowering blood pressure and definitely reducing the levels of hormone cortisol.

From my own personal experience, I can rightly point out that yoga is instrumental in improving the quality of your life by reducing and relieving stress, as well as promoting positive emotions and all forms of positive chemicals and hormones that are required for the body not to wok under stress. Without a doubt, yoga is one of the best ways of relieving stress and ensuring that the body works properly.

Attaining Inner Peace

Yoga is a seamless blend of stretches and exercise along with calming movements that help you to release stress from within your body and mind and to find peace. It's important to focus on your breathing when participating in yoga, this will help to calm and soothe you. When I do yoga, I like to make sure that I am in a quiet environment and that I have enough time to finish a session. You don't need to do a very long session to reap the benefits of relaxation and peace, but you do need to make sure that you are not rushing through it. Be sure to give yourself enough time, you're worth it.

I first started out with yoga in a classroom setting. This was important for me because everyone was learning together and there was a greater connection between us all. You could also start out with books or videos if you are more comfortable alone. Do what feels most comfortable to you. Once you decide how you're going to start doing yoga, push out anything negative that may be bothering you and release it as you exercise.

There are many beginner yoga moves that you can start with. I personally started with very simple ones and focused on my breathing and connecting with myself. This helped me to find peace and to be calm, not only while I was doing the yoga but it carried over with me afterwards. The serene act of the flowing movements and setting out a special quiet time for yourself can help you to take leaps and bounds on your own personal path to inner peace.

A simple pose that I started out with was to sit with my legs crossed, hands on the knees, and thumb and index fingers pinched together. Next, I closed my eyes and focused carefully on my breathing, inhaling the positive and good things and exhaling the negative and stress. It it's difficult for you to stay focused, it's okay. Just pull your thoughts back in and stay on target for at least five minutes. This is a simple and quick relaxation that you can do at any time of the day.

Yoga is ideal for anyone to use. There are many different moves that you can do, if you're looking for stretches to help strengthen your body, you can find it with yoga. If you're intent on losing weight that are also many weight loss yoga moves that you can do as well. The best part of yoga is that while you're attaining inner peace by finding calmness inside of you, you can also make your body stronger. This contributes to your mental wellbeing. When my body feels better, I feel better.

I encourage you to take some time out for yoga today, you'll be amazed at how much more peaceful that you will feel. If you get into the practice of releasing things and taking out quiet time for yourself each day, you will be able to find true inner peace.

Mistakes You Want to Avoid

Yoga can be a great way to stay healthy and strong; however, there are common mistakes that people sometimes make with yoga such as not breathing properly. Yoga breathing should be full-belly breathing. Breathing should be performed by inhaling through your nose and then slowly exhaling through your mouth. Another common mistake is comparing yourself to others during the yoga exercises. Keep in mind; each person learns how to do yoga exercises in their own way. Some learn quicker than others but that doesn't mean that they are performing the exercises better than you. It is important to not compare yourself to others. Simply focus on the routine and how good the exercises will make your feel.

Another mistake some people make with yoga is by coming to class with a full stomach. Yoga, like most exercises, should be done on a somewhat empty stomach. Having too much in your stomach will slow you down, make you feel uncomfortable and leave your muscles short-changed on the energy you need to complete the exercises. Taking the wrong class is another mistake some people make. Those who take an advanced class in yoga but who are not prepared, will not do well because they do not have a good understanding of the different poses that will be performed in that class.

Most importantly, it is always a good idea before starting any yoga class to introduce yourself to the teacher. By talking with the teacher first and letting him or her know that this is your first yoga class and that you are a bit nervous, will help that teacher pay more attention to you, so that you will get the most out of the class. Standing in the wrong spot, is another mistake some early yoga learners make. If you are new to yoga, it is best not to stand in the front line of the class. Those who have taken yoga classes, say that it is better to stand in the middle if you are new, so that you can watch those who are more experienced in front of you. That way you can see how they are doing the exercises.

Wearing clothes that are uncomfortable, clothes that are too baggy, can also be a mistake. Actually, yoga practices go much better when you wear form-fitting clothing. When performing yoga, it is important that you can breathe well as you work out. Loose clothes can get in your face and interfere in forward and backward bends. Another mistake that can occur during yoga is feeling insecure. Keep in mind; no one will be judging you during the class. Everyone there simply wants to do the positions and do well.

There are many benefits of yoga such as: adding more flexibility to your body, obtaining better posture, feeling more relaxed and less stressed and enjoying lower blood pressure. Because yoga is consistent and organized, many feel much calmer during and after the yoga positions. In addition, yoga is also known to lower cholesterol and provide a healthier immune system.

Yoga can also provide strength and endurance benefits.

To conclude, there are various mistakes that some make when starting out with yoga; however, such mistakes can be corrected by continuing the yoga positions. With the many benefits offered from yoga, it just makes sense to check it out! Find out more about yoga and how it can change your life!

Putting It into Action!

Now that you have a general understanding of yoga, it is time to put this into practice. Take action today by joining a yoga class either offered through a local community college or your city's parks and recreation department. Getting started is always the hardest part; it does take courage. But I promise you that once you start everything gets easier. And that is when the fun really begins.

I wish you all the best!

WAIT! Before You Leave…

Download the #1 Bestseller from Gamma Mouse Media for FREE! Hurry this offer won't last as it is for a limited time only. Reserve your free copy today at http://gammamouse.com.

A Special Gift for Our Readers!

Thank you so much for your purchase of this book. As a special gift for you we have included one of our bestselling Self-Improvement books: Procrastination: Triple Your Productivity and Accomplish Your Goals written by one of the most well-respected and influential experts on time management, Warren R. Sullivan.

I hope you enjoy!

Procrastination
Triple Your Productivity and Accomplish Your Goals

Warren R. Sullivan

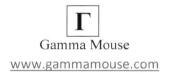

Gamma Mouse
www.gammamouse.com

Introduction

Procrastination. It has a drastic effect on productivity, on our ability to accomplish our goals in life. It can greatly impact our happiness, as we avoid doing something that we are dreading. Yet having to do it still hangs over our head.

Delaying something in order to often do something easier is an easy trap to fall into. Do it enough, and it suddenly becomes a habit. The problem with procrastination is we usually put off more important—but also more difficult—objectives for doing actions that are more trivial. For example, a college student might watch television rather than write a report.

Our time is valuable. It is the one thing that cannot be replaced, unlike money or objects. Yet it is wasted when we procrastinate. Saving this time should be our goal. We need to realize that our time would be better spend on accomplishing our most important objectives. When you have finished those, then reward yourself.

Stopping our procrastination is as easy as changing our attitude and stopping the habit that we have fallen into. In reading this guide, you will learn the tips and tricks necessary to stop procrastinating and start living. You don't have to suffer any longer, you can be happy and more productive, accomplishing all the important goals in your life quickly and easily. But you must take the first step and make a commitment to change yourself. Reading this book is a start, but if you don't act on what you learn change will not come. So consider this a call to action, a chance to truly change your life.

Getting to the root of the problem

Everyone procrastinates. It is part of being human. Whether because of laziness or not having the energy to tackle a difficult task, we choose to relax, to take the easy way out. Understand that not all procrastination should be viewed as bad. Often we need a break from the rigors of our day, a chance to get away from the stress of life. Some goals require great effort and energy to complete, so tackling them when you don't have much energy is realistic.

The line we don't want to cross is when we fool ourselves into believing that laziness is not having the energy to complete our task. Our first step is to recognize when we are being lazy. Clearly, we need to be honest with ourselves, we need to hold ourselves accountable. Secondly, we need to realize that time is our most valuable resource, and that it is finite. No one knows how much time they have, so it is essential to understand how important time is. When you sit down to watch television, recognize that this is time you will never get back.

To borrow a phrase from economics, understand that there is an opportunity cost to ever action you take. When you choose to do something, you lose the opportunity to use that time differently. When you make a choice, there is always a cost, remind yourself of this when you find yourself procrastinating. One of my methods for reminding myself to utilize every minute of my time as effectively as I can is to write the number 1440 on the white board in my office. This is the number of minutes in one day. Whenever I find myself procrastinating, I look at my board, and it helps me refocus on my task at hand.

People procrastinate for different reasons. The first step is to understand the reasoning behind our procrastinating. There may be more than one, but understanding the psychology behind our choices will help us effectively combat them, allowing us to change our faulty reasoning when it arises.

Cognitive distortions are a form of irrational thinking that often lead to procrastination. It is a magically type of thinking. Often we believe that we will be better equipped at some point in the future to handle our task, rather than completely the task at that time.

An example is a person who believes that they need to be in a certain mood in order to complete a task successfully. Or a person may believe that their motivation will increase in the future, and thus will be in a better position to accomplish their goals. Another one that happens in business quite frequently is an employee overestimating the time they have left to complete a task while also underestimating how long it will take them to do it.

If you are putting off a task, because you believe that you will be better suited in the future, realize that you are committing a fallacy. There is no evidence suggesting that your belief is true.

When we are confused about how to complete a task, and the details involved, we may procrastinate giving the reason that we need further instructions before we can continue. This allows us to set the project aside, until we find that we are butting up against a deadline. This reasoning often comes up with perfectionists who do not want to start a task until they are confident in their ability to complete it perfectly. To combat this reasoning, understand that completely the task initially to the best of your abilities and understanding, and then waiting for feedback is much more productive. It is easy to make corrections to your mistakes once the task is completed, as opposed to trying to do the task perfectly the first time. And there is always the possibility that the goal will be accomplished on your first attempt, without the need for further clarification. Don't fool yourself into thinking that if you have additional information, you will be better suited to complete the task. This is a cognitive distortion.

An offshoot of this is avoiding a task because you don't know how it should be done, that you require procedural information. Once again, this reasoning arises most often in the perfectionist, who believes they need to wait for the perfect situation in order to be successful. But look at the great inventors throughout history, who only through trial and error found out how to accomplish something amazing. Imagine if they had waited for the perfect moment, these inventions may never have come into existence. Remember that your goal is to accomplish your task, mistakes that you make can always be corrected. Don't fear failure. Instead, recognize it as an opportunity to learn.

I used to suffer from thinking I needed to take the time, to contemplate and reflect, before beginning a job. What I was doing was procrastinating, convincing myself I needed more information. This was clearly a logical fallacy. Thinking about the job was not going to make me more productive. What was going to make me more productive was doing it. If you believe you need more time to accomplish something, stop and examine whether that is true. Even if it is true, you can start the task now and revise it later as your thoughts begin to coalesce.

We have all had tasks that we had to do that we really didn't want to do. Income taxes come to mind. It is a responsibility, and sometimes that additional pressure makes a task unpleasant. And we are human, we do not want to do things we find unpleasant. We may even fool ourselves into thinking that there will be a point in the future when it will be easier to deal with an unpleasant task. Never make the mistake to think that a task that is unpleasant today will somehow miraculously improve in the future. It is always better to get the unpleasantness over immediately, rather than wait. I am reminded of my public speaking class in college. I always wanted to go first, and I could never understand why people wouldn't want to be first. Most found public speaking uncomfortable and unpleasant, but instead of immediately getting it out of the way and then relaxing, they chose to prolong how long the task would take them. Don't fall victim to this. If you find a task unpleasant, do it immediately; procrastination only makes it worse, and in the process makes you unhappy.

Now the opposite of procrastinating over tasks that we find unpleasant is to procrastinate over accomplishing goals that we don't care about. Finding the effort to complete a task when you are indifferent to the outcome is difficult. Often we may believe that we will feel more inclined to complete a task in the future when we feel more connected with the outcome. Usually indifference does not change, people don't suddenly start to care. These types of tasks often don't get tackled until we run up against a deadline. This can cause us additional stress as we must now take time to complete a task we don't care about instead of tasks that are much more important to us. Understand the cost of procrastinating may not be felt until the future when the task must be completed. Completing the task immediately saves you from future repercussions that you cannot anticipate.

I previously relayed the example of people believing that at some point in the future they will be in a better mood to accomplish a task. They may believe that certain moods make them more productive and believe that they need to wait for when they are in that mood. Recognize that this is an irrational reason you are giving yourself in order to procrastinate. While your emotions can affect your work, this is only generally in the case of extremes. Slight fluctuations in mood will have no effect, so don't convince yourself that you will be in a better mood to complete the task in the future. There is no truth to this.

A more specific example of this idea that a certain mood is essential for higher productivity is the case of individuals who wait until the last moment to start a task. The student who begins to study for mid-terms the night before the text, or the employee who starts an project the day before it is due are two examples of this. Waiting until the last minute to start because you think you are more productive up against a deadline is nothing more than believing that your mood makes you more productive at a point in the future. Don't fall for this procrastination excuse.

An additional reason you don't want to wait until you are up against a deadline is the cognitive distortion in which you overestimate the time you have while underestimating how long it will take you to accomplish a task. If you wait, believing you work better under pressure, you may place yourself in a situation in which you have significantly underestimated the time you will need. This may cause you to rush, resulting in sub-standard work. Or, even worse, you may miss your deadline completely. Avoid backing yourself into this corner where time works against you. Remember that we often believe that we have more time than we actually do.

Another reason people often give for procrastinating is that they had forgotten about a job. Often the reason that it was forgotten is intentional, the task may be unpleasant or one that we are indifferent about. If a deadline is far into the future, it can be easy to forget about our upcoming responsibilities. Or we may believe that we will get to it closer to the deadline. Understand that this is procrastination, and that there is nothing keeping you from completing the job now.

The final cognition distortion I will address is the belief that you don't want to currently complete a job because you are not feeling well, and that you will wait until you feel better. It should be evident how this is very similar to waiting for a specific mood in order to complete a task. Understand that there is no guarantee that you will feel better, in fact, you may end up feeling worse. Granted that people suffer from real health problems that greatly impact their ability to be productive. This is not what I am referring to. Instead, I refer to procrastinators who exaggerate how they feel to shirk their responsibilities. Don't be disingenuous with yourself about how you feel in order to avoid doing something.

Many of these cognition distortions are rooted in perfectionism or in our fear. We are either waiting for the moment to be right, or we are waiting to overcome our fear to do a task we may find unpleasant. Tell yourself that the moment will never be perfect, but it will be good enough to get the job done. Or if you are dealing with fear, realize that confronting your fear and doing the job now, will mean that once you have finished you will no longer have anything to fear. In fact, you will likely feel elated. This is a much better situation to be in than living under a cloud of dread.

Now that we have explored the underlying psychological reasons behind procrastination, our attention will turn to effective methods for dealing with procrastination. By employing the appropriate methods to our life, we will be able to become happier and more productive people.

Recognize the problem

Like with any addiction or problem, the first step is always to recognize and accept that you have a problem. Since you have purchased this book, I will assume that you have identified yourself as a procrastinator, and are now taking the proper steps to remedy this.

Do not feel shamed or embarrassed, identifying and attacking your problems is a noble and brave action. Focus on your self-awareness; stopping procrastination means keeping a keen eye on your behaviors. And making the necessary corrections.

Exercise

I want you to exam your behavior and thought processes. Write down three incidents in which you procrastinated.

Refer to the previous chapter if you want to show why your reasoning was faulty.

Find the root of the problem

Why are you procrastinating? Are you a perfectionist? Is fear keeping you from accomplishing certain tasks? Be honest with yourself. Discovering the root of your procrastination is important. If you recognize the cognition distortions that you are employing, this will give you a hint at the root of your procrastination. While knowing the underlying cause is helpful, identifying your faulty reasoning so you can correct it will have greater long-term gains.

If you are a perfectionist or if fear is holding you back, I want you to take a moment and examine your thinking. Why do you have to be perfect? Does it make you more productive? Does it make you happier? My guess is the answer will be "no". Tell yourself that accomplishing something perfectly is not the goal, the goal is only accomplishing your task. Withhold judgment, jobs are either done or not done. Also, ask yourself is it true that the longer you wait, the closer you will be to perfect? Or would you have done the same job either way? Does the evidence actually support your way of thinking?

The same approach can be taken if you suffer from fear. Ask yourself what you are afraid of? Most people fear a specific outcome. Is it rational to believe that outcome is guaranteed? I may fear dying in a plane crash, so I dread getting on a plane. But what are the chances that this event actually occurs. My chances are much greater of dying in a car accident on the way to the airport, but I don't have the same dread getting into a car. By nature, fear is not rational; it often arises from the fact that we have convinced ourselves of a terrible outcome, even though that outcome may be incredibly remote. Try to look at your fear rationally; assess the likelihood of the outcomes you fear. Then ask yourself: is it really that bad? Surprisingly, our fears are often overstated; they have a tendency to shrink when we look at them rationally.

Exercise

Using the previous chapter, identify any cognitive distortions you have fallen victim to. Can you discern what is behind this? If it is fear or the desire to be perfect, look at potential outcomes. Does it really need to be perfect? Is it a situation that you should be fearful of? Write down the reasons why you believe you need to be perfect, or write down why you should be afraid. Put it away for a day, and then read it again. Do your thoughts appear logical?

Prioritize with lists

Writing down a list is very effective in helping you achieve your goals. But you need to stick with it. Many people write lists, and then don't follow them. Remember the list is to help you stop procrastinating. Once you write the list, don't convince yourself out of following the order you set.

Put the jobs in order of priority, the most important being first and the least important being last. Estimate how long you believe each task will take you. Then multiply that time by a factor of three. Set this revised time as your deadline. The extra time will take into account the possibility that you are underestimating how long each task will take you; it serves as a buffer. The benefit is that if you complete your tasks early, you now have that extra time to do things you want to.

Keep your list close at hand. You can either write it down, or like I do, keep it on a mobile device.

There are numerous to-do list apps that will simplify the process.

Exercise

Write a list in which you prioritize your tasks by level of importance. Decide how long it will take you to do each task, then multiply that number by three. Write down the time needed next to each task on your list.

Divide and conquer

There are some tasks that are so large and unwieldy that estimating how long they will take is an incredibly difficult job. To help facilitate the process, break the large job into smaller segments. These segments should be small enough that you can estimate the time each one of them will take. Make certain you add in a buffer by multiplying each estimated time by three.

If you have a specific deadline, you can now add the time estimations for each of the smaller tasks to arrive at a figure for the entire project. This is a fantastic way to estimate large projects without placing yourself in a stressful situation as the deadline approaches. In fact, this approach is used quite frequently in the software industry for large multi-team projects.

Exercise

If you have a large project on your list, particularly if you are having difficulty estimating how long it will take, break it down into smaller segments. Now evaluate how much time each task will take, keeping the added buffer in mind.

Keep distractions to a minimum

One of the biggest productivity killers in recent years for businesses has been the Internet. It becomes easier for employees to procrastinate when they have other options that are more appealing only a mouse click away. With social media and email, there is always something new happening, and it can be quite difficult not to get immersed in this flow of constant information.

There are productivity plugins that will limit your access to the Internet by allowing you to stay online for short periods of time. If possible, I also recommend shutting down your email program, and only checking it at designated times. One method that is effective is to focus on your task for the first 50 minutes in the hour. In the remaining ten minutes, you can then check your email or Facebook status.

Additionally, a work or home environment can be distracting. People talking, a television playing, and other background noise can make you lose your focus. Listening to music through headphones or using earplugs is effective in blocking out distracting noise.

Exercise

Are you being distracted? Analyze your environment and decide whether you are being distracted. If you find yourself going online to check email or surf the Internet, try to use the 50 minute rule. Browser plugins will also limit your access to the Internet. Research, install, and configure them if you need this level of restriction.

If noise is a problem, buy earplugs or bring your headphones and MP3 player in order to listen to music.

Celebrate your accomplishments

You have completed your task list; time to celebrate. Giving yourself a reward after accomplishing your goals is wonderful way to encourage yourself to leave procrastination behind. The reward can be anything, an hour of television, a movie and dinner out, or an item you want. The point is to make it something you really desire, to properly give you a sense of accomplishment.

Exercise

Schedule a reward for yourself for completing your task list. Make it good. You deserve it.

Take care of yourself

Eating right and sleeping the recommended amount by your physician is essential in helping to reduce stress and anxiety. It is much easier to tackle your task list if you are feeling energized after a good night's sleep followed by a substantial breakfast. Often poor eating habits during the day lead to your blood sugar crashing in the afternoon, leaving you feeling sluggish and tired.

Make a point of eating a balanced diet spread over at least three meals over the course of the day. Maintain a regimented sleeping schedule. Try to go to bed and wake up at approximately the same time every day. Maintaining our sleep rhythms is very important.

Exercise, put it as a high priority on your task list if you have to. This can be as simple as taking a short walk. Exercising has the wonderful effect of increasing your energy, so take advantage.

Exercise

Evaluate your eating and sleeping habits, making the necessary changes. If you are not exercising, start. It can be as simple as a thirty minute walk per day.

Learn to say no

Many of us have the tendency to want to please other people. We take on more tasks and responsibilities than we have time for, causing us to have too many things to accomplish and not enough time to do them in. If you become too overwhelmed, there is a very good chance you will procrastinate rather than tackle your enormous list.

Learning to say no to task of low importance is key. When someone asks you to do something, look at what they are asking objectively. Is this task a high priority to you? What is the opportunity cost to you? Remember that your time is extremely valuable, it cannot be replaced. Time you spend on this task could be spent elsewhere. Unless it is a close family member, the most time I'm willing to spend on a task for someone is ten minutes. If I don't think I can accomplish it in ten minutes (after adding in my buffer), I will apologize and tell the person that I can't do it. Most people understand, they realize that we all lead busy lives. And if they don't, it is only further justification that I made the right decision.

Exercise

Look at your task list. Are there low priority jobs on it that you agreed to do for other people? If so, remove them from your list and let the person know, unless you believe you can accomplish it in a very short timeframe.

Be proactive in obtaining the information you need

During our examination of cognition distortions, we talked about procrastinating because we lack specific information about how to proceed or what our ultimate goal was. The way to avoid this problem is to always ask questions immediately on being given the task. Make certain you understand what your deliverables will be as well as the best way to proceed. There is no harm in asking and getting the answer. It will save you both time and aggravation.

With the advent of cellphones and email, people are generally accessible within a few hours. If the person you need to ask is not available, try to ask someone who has completed a similar task. Asking questions is not only an effective method for curtailing procrastination, it also has a generally positive affect on your life. We live in a society where the majority of people ask too few questions.

Exercise

Examine your task list. Is there a task that you have questions about? If so, contact the person who can answer your questions immediately. Even if it is late, send them an email. Don't wait, act on your questions right now.

Get into the habit

Procrastination is a bad habit, emphasis on habit. Habits need to be broken, and the best way to accomplish this is by replacing them with a new habit. If you have taken the suggested action to this point, you have already started on your way to replacing your habit to procrastinate. But it is only the start. Generally, it is believed that if a person can change their behavior for twenty-one days that change will become permanent.

Exercise

Find a calendar and mark off twenty-one days from today. Your goal is to keep up on doing your task list daily for the twenty-one days. Be aware that you will have to fight to keep procrastination from coming back in. Replacing old habits can be difficult, which means you need to remain vigilant of any back-sliding.

Make tasks relevant to you

Many of the jobs we do are done despite us being indifferent to the task or not enjoying it. The easiest way to combat this is to look at the task and accentuate a positive aspect of it. If you can find a good reason for doing something, it will make accomplishing it much more attractive to you. Think outside the box for reasons if you have to. Maybe completing a task will open up a new opportunity in your life, or allow you to connect with different people. Accomplishing it may give you the opportunity to make new friends.

There are a variety of reasons why a task should be completed. You need to find the one that holds the most appeal to you.

Exercise

Take a moment to examine your list. Are there any jobs you do not enjoy to do? Are there any tasks you feel indifferent about? If so, think of a good reason, one that appeals to you, of what completing the task could mean for you. Try to find a reason that makes you want to tackle the job.

Conclusion

I hope that you have found this journey helpful. If you have participated in the recommended exercises along the way, you should be commended. You have clearly decided you want to change, and that is a huge first step to becoming a more productive person.

Procrastination is not something you need to suffer with, the answers are all right here in this guide. Understand that procrastination can have deep psychological roots, causes that take time and effort to overcome. The best way to accomplish this is to face it head on. If you are a perfectionist, try completing a task even though you may not feel it is perfect, or up to your usual standards. If fear is holding you back, stand up to it by imagining the worst outcome, and then honestly evaluating how likely that outcome will come to be.

Humans suffer from many irrational thoughts, convinced of the truth of an idea even though the evidence suggests the opposite. Recognizing these irrational thoughts is the first step in dispelling them. Once you realize you are being illogical, the thought fails to hold any power over you anymore. Never take anything for granted, continuously question your thoughts, assessing them for validity. This isn't only the key to stopping procrastination, it also leads to a life that is happier and more productive.

I wish you all the success in your journey.

WAIT! Before You Leave…

Download the #1 Bestseller from Gamma Mouse Media for FREE! Hurry this offer won't last as it is for a limited time only. Reserve your free copy today at http://gammamouse.com.